The Thyroid [

By

Lynne D M Noble

Independently published 2023

About the Author

Lynne Noble was born in 1953 in Huddersfield, West Yorkshire. From a very early age, Lynne showed an interest in nutrition and genetics avidly reading any books that she could get her hands on at the time.

Initially, Lynne studied orthopaedics but events led her to work with the elderly mentally infirm. Here, her interest in neurodegenerative disorders and pain syndromes developed.

Lynne undertook rigorous programmes of study, completing her Cert Ed., (FE) BSc (Hons) and Adv. Dip Education simultaneously before moving onto her M.Ed.

From there she took further demanding programmes in Human Nutrition, Pharmacology, Neuroscience, Genetics and Immunology. During this time, she was given many prestigious awards for her academic work. It was noted then that Lynne was not afraid of tackling difficult subjects.

She began her law degree but ill health prevented her from pursuing this. However, in this time, she moved from being a foster parent to adoptive parent.

She has been instrumental in setting up projects in the community for disadvantaged groups.

She is a member of the Guild of Health Writers and the British Union of Journalists.

Now retired, she lives with her husband in a historic Georgian riverside town in the West Midlands. She enjoys gardening, watching her husband bowling and researching.

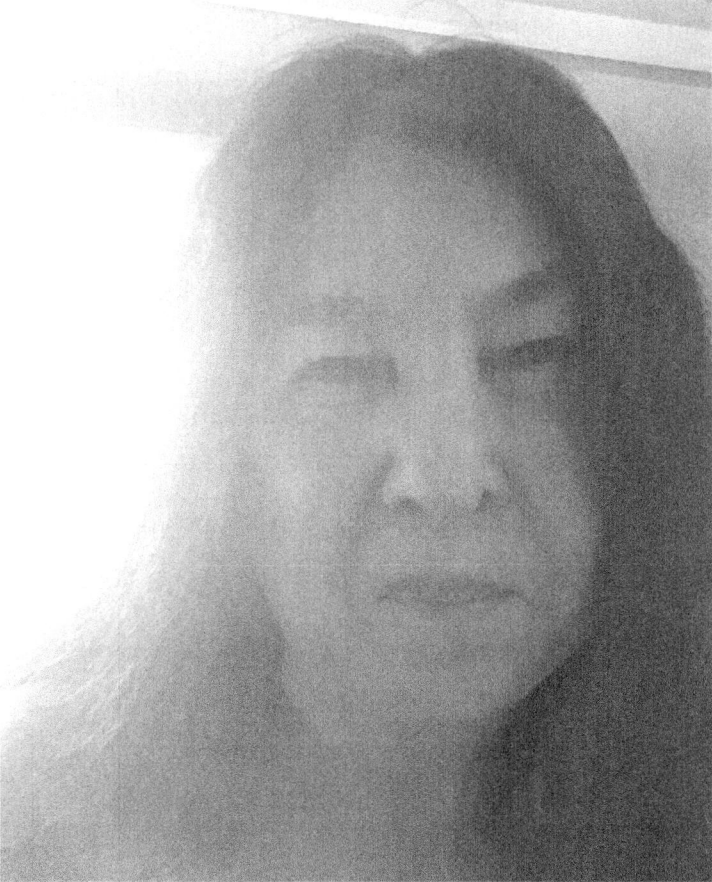

Author Lynne Noble, aged 67 years, at home

https://quintessentiallylynne.weebly.com/nutritional-medicine.html

Table of contents

With special thanks to @KazNan3 for her support of my work.

Preface

I understand that there is a great deal of frustration from those who suffer from thyroid disorders and who wish to get off their thyroid medication. There appears to be little help out there for them apart from books repeating over and over again what goes wrong with thyroid function. The punchline then is 'and the treatment is thyroxine, for life.'

I am not – and have never been – a great believer that any medication should be for life where someone has not been born with a condition. Any condition that manifests itself in later life occurs as a result of something happening in the body which, for example, could be a deficiency, an excess or an infection or injury. This is not a definitive list. The point I am trying to make is that it has occurred because of a new situation and, if this is the case – and the new situation can be identified that is causing thyroid function to go awry - then it can be addressed and reversed.

Reversal is not always easy. It may require a great deal of investigation. The body is a wonderfully complex piece of machinery and what we think is going wrong may be a few steps removed from what is *actually* going on.

When we consider dietary deficiencies it is hard to believe that in what is one of the richest countries in the world, deficiencies can and do occur.

Deficiencies, however, can be due to the lack of availability of foods which provide the nutrient in question or that the nutrient is found in only a few foods. Vitamin D is a case of the latter and unless you live in a country where there are good amounts of sunshine daily then it is quite likely that a deficiency of vitamin D exists.

Some foods labelled as being high in a nutrient – brazils nuts are noted for containing selenium, may not contain anywhere near the amount you would expect if they are grown in selenium depleted soils.

Some nutrients are quite vulnerable and are easily degraded. The B vitamins are easily destroyed by heat or light and, as they are water soluble, anything boiled will leach the B vitamins into the water. This is generally thrown away.

In some cases, the recommended daily amount of a specific nutrient may be eaten but nutrients may not be absorbed without other nutrients being present. For example, iron needs vitamin C in order for it to be bioavailable. Vitamin D needs magnesium in order for it to be activated.

Other deficiencies occur due to the numerous food fads that abound at the moment. Any food group taken out of the diet does not provide for a well-balanced diet. Carbohydrates are demonised, animal fats are demonised. Meat is out of favour. Apparently, only plant milks are suitable for humans without any thought of the anti-nutrients which inhibit vital nutrients.

Pharmaceutical medications may inhibit nutrients. Metformin, for example, degrades thiamine, an absolutely vital nutrient which impacts every cell in the body.

Just as a deficiency should concern us – and goes largely unrecognised -   an excess of nutrients can also impact our health and the ability of our organs to function correctly.

The excess does not have to occur because of a greatly increased intake of food. The current scourge is an excessive intake of supplements which has now become just as alarming as the enthusiastic prescribing of drugs for some ailments which would settle down fairly quickly if left.

Zinc, whilst it has enormous potential for health is able, if taken in excessive quantities, to inhibit the absorption of copper and iron thus contributing to a deficiency of these trace minerals.

Recently, in communication with someone on social media, I found out that their daily supplement intake was:

Ashwaganda

Iodine

Vitamin D

Vitamin C

Gingko biloba

Curcumin

L-theanine

Soya milk shakes

Zinc

Allicin

Quercetin

Magnesium

Calcium

The individual mentioned that they suffered from anxiety but this was obvious from the inclusion of the above into their daily supplements which to say was excessive, was probably an understatement.

I only ever recommend supplements where there is a known cause and reason to include supplements as a therapeutic response to a known condition.

The only supplement that I recommend that everyone take most of the year round is vitamin D3 because it is available in such few foods. Yes, you can take a break from it during the summer months on very sunny days but other than that, it should be your main, if not your only, supplement.

As you age, you may have to consider further nutrients to supplement as absorption of nutrients is not as effective once you reach the age of 50.

Older people get to the stage where they cannot eat in the same quantity as they could when they were younger. This has the effect of limiting the nutrients that they eat. Smaller, more nutritionally dense meals, will largely address this life stage.

Some supplementation is based on very limited knowledge, something that has been researched or heard from another but which is not really sound information.

However, this book is about those who have hypothyroidism or Hashimoto's disease and how such conditions may due to nutritional deficiencies which can by replacing the missing nutrients, be reversed.

Modern medicine tends not to focus on a cure or reversal of a condition. This book, however, is different. My focus is always on correcting the underlying cause of the condition rather than addressing the symptoms.

Thyroid Disease- A background

Hashimoto's disease is an autoimmune disorder. The immune system creates antibodies that attack the cells of the thyroid gland. The antibodies do not recognise the thyroid cell as being part of its system, it sees it as foreign and calls for some immune system cells to deal with them.

Tiny cells they might be but immune system cells have a range of defences which can pack a powerful punch. When you have an infection, it is not the infective agent that causes the pain, it is the immune system going into all-out war against what it perceives to be the enemy.

Eventually, the thyroid becomes so damaged that it is unable to work properly. Initially the symptoms may be vague. The patient may complain of tiredness, weight gain and muscle weakness. The symptoms may be attributed to the menopause or something else going on in the individual's life. The enlarged thyroid gland manifests itself later.

Hypothyroidism occurs when the thyroid gland makes insufficient thyroid hormone. The condition is also referred to as an underactive thyroid.

This is a condition that develops slowly over many years and is unlikely to be noticed in its early stages. If it isn't treated, then high cholesterol and heart problems may occur.

Diagnosis of hypothyroidism is through a blood test and if positive then thyroid hormones are prescribed.

As with Hashimoto's disease, initial symptoms are fatigue and weight gain. However, the metabolism will continue to slow down and produce symptoms, some of which are associated with a poorly functioning thyroid. These include:

Sensitivity to cold (a well-recognised symptom)

fatigue

weight gain

dry, puffy skin

constipation

stiff, aching muscles and muscle weakness

coarse hair and skin

hoarse voice

thinning hair

bradycardia (slower than normal heart rate)

cognitive disorders

mood disorders such as depression

Now, I must return to the subject of excess supplementation and our penchant for supplementing with iodine for one reason for the problems we have with the thyroid.

However, we will take a mini look at thyroid hormones and medications first although most people with thyroid problems are well acquainted with the terminology.

Thyroid hormones, active, inactive, man-made or not

There are two main thyroid hormones in the body which help regulate metabolism including the regulation of body temperature, the metabolic rate of digestive, heart function and bone maintenance among others. These hormones are referred to as T3 - which is the active form - and T4 which is the largely inactive form.

Once the thyroid releases the inactive T4 it is transformed into T3 so that it can impact cells. Uptake of T3 is improved by the addition of fats (not seed oils which are inflammatory in nature). Cell receptors are abler to take up thyroid hormones as they are lipid soluble. Those on low fat diets are at a disadvantage.

When our own thyroid hormones are lacking then meds will be prescribed. No investigations regarding diet or other potential causes will be undertaken. No, the hormone levels will be determined and a medication prescribed. The patient will be told that it will be for the rest of their life. Not an exciting prospect.

The two synthetic hormones are Levothyroxine (Synthroid) which is a synthetic form of T4 and Cytomel (liothyronine) which is a synthetic form of T3.

Normally, T4 is prescribed. The reasons for this is that it has a longer half-life. This is true but the conversion of T4 to T3 may be problematical and I have known of people who have been prescribed Levothyroxine when the problem was T3 based - in that the conversion from T4 to T3 was the difficulty that would not be solved by the above prescribing measures.

One lady's experience of misprescribing was:

'If only I could have the energy to write about the 25 years they #NHS mistreated my low #thyroid (gave me levothyroxine) kept giving it to me even though it didn't work (I needed #T3) I was falling asleep when driving – GP said, 'You must be bored.'

Another stated:

I have subclinical hypothyroidism that doctors won't treat in spite of me having had symptoms so I just started taking nascent iodine and am doing well on that. My eyebrows even started growing back. Doctors live and die by lab #s, not symptoms.

I shall return to this subject later as clearly we need to know about the conversion process of the thyroxine hormones and any inhibitors of the process other than a low fat diet.

In contrast, iodine is water soluble. We are well acquainted with the knowledge that too little iodine is a risk factor for thyroid problems but can an excess of iodine also create problems?

It is to this subject that we now turn.

Excessive Iodine and Hashimoto's Disease

Iodine is a mineral found in some foods. Iodine is needed to synthesise thyroid hormones which direct the pace of the body's metabolism among many other important functions.

In order to test for thyroid levels in your blood Thyroid Stimulating Hormones (TSH) are measured. If your levels of thyroid hormones are too low, then the pituitary gland picks this up and makes larger amounts of TSH. This instructs your thyroid gland to work a little harder. The pituitary is also able to put a brake on TSH when it detects that there is too much thyroid hormone. Thus, the measurement of TSH is used by medics to decide whether there is a problem with the thyroid gland which needs addressing. Of course, this assumes that all individuals will fall neatly into an arbitrary reference range when clearly, individuals are far too complex to be shunted into a convenient box.

Listening to people's stories has been an uncomfortable one for me for the pain, frustration and suffering that they have endured is very real.

Can I say how dismissive healthcare practitioners are about this subject. Following my diagnosis every time, I needed to see my GP regarding another matter, I was told my thyroid was causing it.

Dawn

Adults require 150mcg of iodine daily. Pregnant women need slightly more with the recommended daily intake of 220mcg.

Many foods provide iodine including:

Fish

Dairy products which includes milk and cheese

Eggs

Iodised salt

Vegetarian sources include:

 Wholegrains

Seaweed

Spring greens

Beans

Courgettes

Prunes

watercress

However, food analyses are virtually meaningless as the food content of iodine depends on the soil content of food.

Worldwide distribution varies a great deal. The 'goitre belt' refers to any area lacking the mineral iodine.

In the UK the 'goitre belt' is the Midlands and South West England. In the USA it stretches across the middle of the country.

For those who are relying on obtaining this mineral from locally grown produce they will not obtain enough and may have to supplement with iodine.

Most of the iodine that we have is concentrated in the thyroid gland. However, a little is found in serum as T3 (triiodothyronine) and T4 (thyroxine).

The functions of T3 and T4 are simple in that they are responsible for the rate of metabolism in the body and for converting food into energy.

However, it is not just a case of dietary iodine ensuring the proper function of the thyroid gland. The thyroid gland performs functions which include detoxification, calcium homeostasis, the regulation of the cellular metabolic rate among many others.

A deficiency of iodine is associated with iron deficiency, depression and anxiety. It is also associated with autism.

We shall look at the hypothyroid patient shortly but it is also helpful to look at an alternative view of the causes of the main cause of autoimmune thyroid dysfunction.

In his [1]book *The Thyroid Reset Diet: Reverse Hypothyroidism and Hashimoto's Symptoms with a Proven Iodine Balancing Plan* by Alan Christianson NMD, he proposes that the cause of

Autoimmune thyroiditis was due to too much iodine. Initially, people feel better on additional iodine but then the body begins to fight back against the additional hormones.

There are many nutrients that work within a fairly narrow range and supplementing may tip susceptible people over the limit resulting in autoimmunity.

This makes complete sense to me since while supplements can address many issues, the belief that 'more is better' is something I have witnessed time and time again.

---

[1] Available on Amazon

The other difficulty that I witness is that because a supplement like vitamin D is useful because it is so improbable – if not impossible - to take in enough through diet alone, then all the other nutrients which vitamin D generally works alongside must also be a deficiency risk and therefore must be supplemented. This is far from the case. Young, healthy people are unlikely to be deficient in vitamin K2, this being a vitamin which is made in the gastrointestinal tract. I have never known a young adult be deficient in vitamin K2 yet so it does not require supplementing. It just gives the body more work to do dealing with an excess.

With regards to iodine, many multivitamins do contain excessive doses of iodine. If you add that to the average amount that you take in through food and iodised salt, and that which is added to prepared foods in the form of carrageen, for example, then you can see how easy it is for the balance of iodine – and its impact on the human body – to be tipped out of kilter.

24

The only way through this is to look at your average daily intake through supplements, diet and dietary additions. More is not always better.

Kelp is a popular food for some who are trying to increase their iodine intake. Sometimes the intention is not to increase dietary iodine but merely to have a 'healthy' green smoothie.'

Unfortunately, dried kelp contains 535mcg per gram.

Haddock contains 659mcg per 100g, add this to a latte 130mcg containing a mugful of milk (300ml) and we are way over the recommended daily intake of iodine by far.

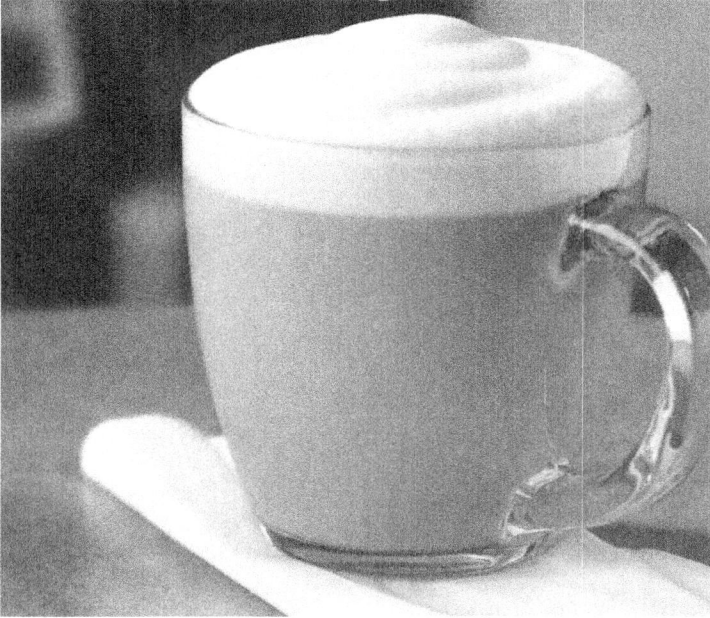

300ml of latte contain nearly the recommended daily intake of iodine.

When I look at dietary books about iodine from decades ago, excess is never a problem. They run along the lines…. excess *is*

unlikely to happen under <u>*normal*</u> *circumstances but may occur in medical treatment…….*

to which I could add supplementation as a contemporary medical treatment with the potential for negative side effects.

Further, our diets have become full of excess. Eating patterns have changed a great deal from the 1950's when carbohydrate fuelled diets were not in evidence in the way that they are now.

Carrageenan is also added to many foods. Although carrageenan – which is a natural ingredient found in red seaweed – only contains small amounts of iodine, it adds up given the numerous products which contains it.

Carrageenan is an additive which is used to emulsify or thicken foods and drinks. It is used in vegan and vegetarian food as a replacement for gelatine.

Carrageen is often added to nut milks, faux meat products and, as a thickener in yogurt.

There are a number of concerns surrounding the detrimental effects that carrageen may have on health.

Evidence suggests that this additive may trigger gastritis, gastric ulceration and other inflammatory disorders like colitis, colon cancer, irritable bowel syndrome, glucose intolerance and bloating, as well as food allergies.

Once a chronic inflammatory reaction is initiated then it may initiate conditions such arthritis or indeed any condition which ends in 'itis' which, of course, just means 'inflammation.'

Indeed, another 'itis' is cholecystitis which is a fancy way of saying 'gallbladder inflammation.'

I add this one – even though it appears entirely unrelated to anything to do with the thyroid' because time and time again when I come across people with thyroid problems they also appear to have – or have had – problems with their gall bladder. When it happens enough times you have to think whether there is a connection or not.

So maybe some of the problems that people have with an inflamed thyroid that is a little out of control may indirectly have something to do with an ingredient added to many foods which not only contains iodine but has an inflammatory component to it.

Chronic inflammation nibbles away at tissue, eventually destroying so much that it is unable to do its job.

As well as the foods already mentioned as containing carrageen, milk shakes, cream, cottage cheese and ice cream, all contain it, too.

Degraded carrageenan has been stated to be the problem but food grade carrageenan has been found to contain a percentage of the degraded form. In addition, there appears to be very little difference between the food grade and degraded forms.

Autoimmunity is the cause of most thyroid conditions. Normally found as Hashimoto's thyroiditis, the immune system goes into overdrive attacking and destroying its own thyroid tissue that it no longer recognises as being self.

Perhaps, just perhaps, our current culture of adding unusual substances to ready foods to make them more appealing and our readiness to supplement isolated nutrients without really understanding the impact of doing so is behind the rapidly growing manifestations of thyroid disorders in our society.

We do have to consider an exhausted thyroid damaged by the relentless feeding of iodine beyond its capabilities to deal with it. Just like an exhausted individual, worked beyond their strength or capabilities, they will stop functioning or function less well. So, there is a 2 stage process here. The overfeeding of the thyroid beyond its means to cope and then following on from that, thyroid gland inflammation, auto immunity and thyroid cancer all of which are associated with high iodine intakes. Really, when inflammatory processes are initiated then they tend to turn into a chronic inflammation as ageing progresses and there is no doubt that thyroid issues are associated with older people.

Of course, when the thyroid is damaged it is unable to make thyroid hormones so metabolic processes slow down; weight gain, feeling cold, brain fog, gastrointestinal problems and all the other myriad of processes that the thyroid hormones are involved with, slow down.

Could the cause of autoimmune thyroiditis be associated with excess iodine? Only withdrawing external sources found in ready foods, iodised salt and supplements may provide the answer.

However, we know that higher intakes of iodine can have symptoms which are not immediately relatable to an iodine excess. These include a metallic taste in the mouth, a burning mouth, stomach upset, a sore throat and sore teeth and gums.

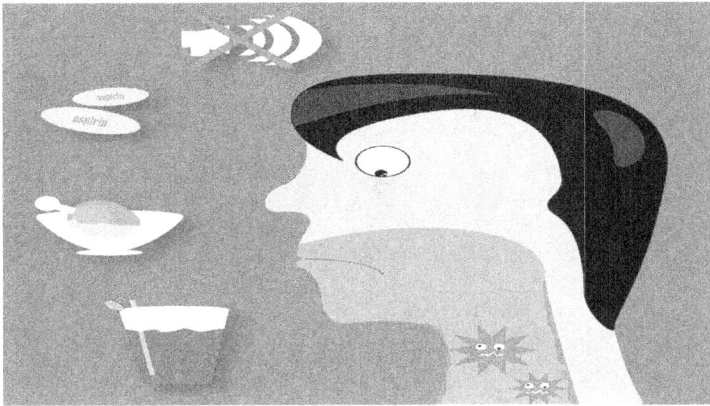

A sore throat may be an indication of excess iodine in the diet

 If the iodine intake is more excessive then nausea and vomiting can also occur. Sometimes it is also a cause of hepatic steatosis.

Hepatic steatosis is an unpleasant condition with equally unpleasant symptoms which include

Abdomen swollen with fluid (ascites)

Enlarged blood vessels just below the skin's surface

Jaundice (the skin and eyes will appear yellow)

Reddening of the palms (beefy palms)

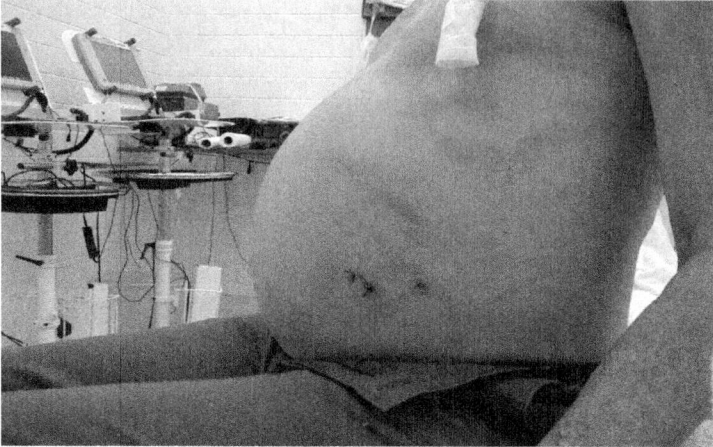

Ascites may be caused by excessive iodine

Before we consider bombarding our bodies with iodine we ought to consider the adage:

The only difference between a medicine and a poison is the dose.

On many occasions, patients are given a package of meds in order to **avoid** a condition, that may or may not occur in the future, is madness. The giving of medicine when none is currently required is equivalent to poisoning someone. They simply do not need it so prescribe such is akin to overdosing.

Dr Izabella Wentz[2] has pointed out that

'excessive doses of iodine can trigger (and worsen) Hashimoto's in people who are genetically predisposed to Hashimoto's and may have certain 'vulnerabilities' such as a selenium deficiency.

Further, temporary iodine restriction may actually improve and even normalise thyroid function, in some individuals.'

Another weapon at our disposal when it comes to thyroid antibodies is that of the supplement myo-inositol. Inositol is also known as vitamin B8 but, for some reason, is rarely included in the B complex supplements. Sometimes it is referred to as lipotropic factor. Lipotropic means the breakdown of fat in which it can be used better for functions in the body and energy.

Inositol is a water soluble nutrient but is not always classed as a true vitamin as the body can make some itself but only in limited quantities.

---

[2] https://thyroidpharmacist.com/articles/iodine-hashimotos/

Most inositol can be found in the brain, kidney, spleen, stomach, heart and liver.

Inositol mainly functions as an anxiolytic and a fat solubilising agent but it also is known to maintain healthy hair as well as controlling blood cholesterol levels.

Sometimes it is used with vitamin E where it is known to restore nerve damage. It also has application in the condition, schizophrenia.

The supplement myo-inositol has been found to reduce thyroid antibody and TSH levels and has a positive impact on mood for thyroid dysfunction is often accompanied by mood swings, anxiety and depressive states. Even Obsessive Compulsive Disorder is associated with a deficiency of this nutrient Additionally, insulin resistance and weight gain are characteristics of a deficiency of myo-inositol as is acne.

Good food sources are:

Wholemeal bread

Green leafy vegetables

Pulses

Molasses

Beef heart

Desiccated liver

Cereals

Steak

Nuts

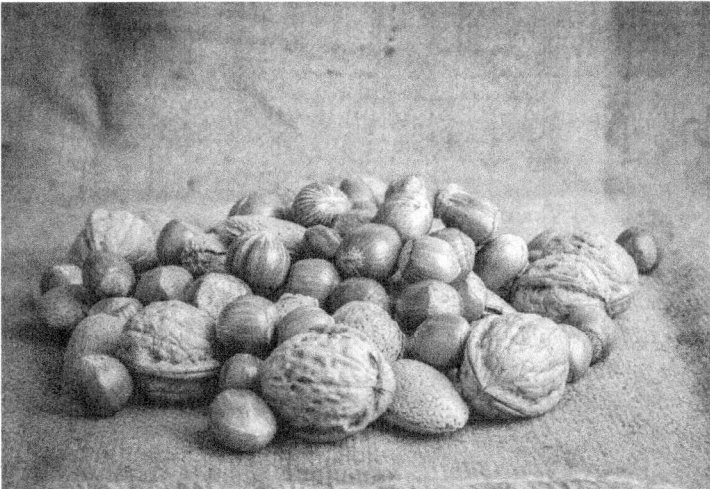

Nuts are a great source of inositol

Inositol is found in cereals where combined with phosphorus it is known as phytic acid. Phytic acid can be a problem insomuch it may inhibit the absorption of some **minerals** such as zinc which is vital for thyroid processes. However, it does not impact **vitamin** uptake.

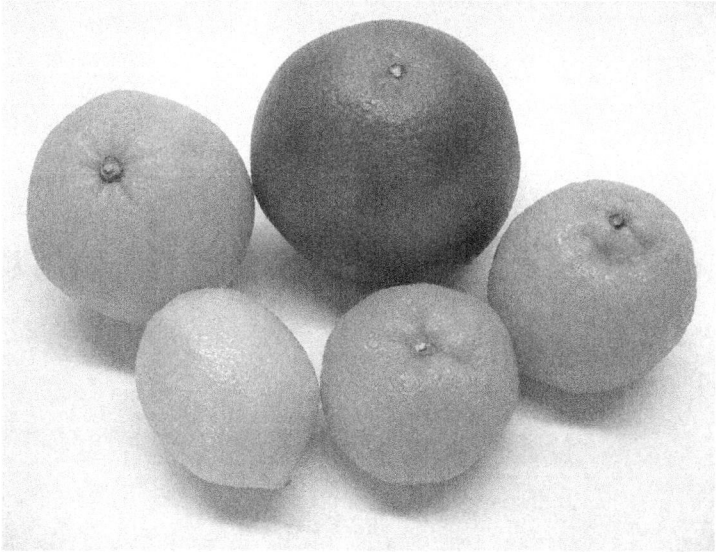

Citrus fruits contain inositol

Of course, there are other risk factors for thyroid disease. We have introduced many medications into our population which impact the way the thyroid works and we shall look at this later.

However, we need to turn our attention to the many new diets that have infiltrated our culture. These includes the explosion of plant based diets, low fat or no fat diets (why?) all of which impact a gland which requires a well-balanced diet in order to function properly. It is not possible to take food groups out and expect to remain healthy because this may deprive a metabolic pathway of the means to complete its function. Younger people appear to get away with this but this neglect of the requirements of the human body will catch up with them later.

Fats are extremely important in the diet but unfortunately saturated fat found in foods of animal origin have been demonised. This is regrettable. Unlike the seed oils – sunflower oil for example – which cause highly inflammatory processes in the body, saturated fat cannot and does not.

When something is saturated it is akin to a group of children all holding each other's hands. They do not have spare hands in which to get up to mischief or, as we say in scientific terms, react with anything.

The seed oils, however, ARE reactive. They are like a group of children where a pair refuse to hold hands. Those spare hands are ready to get up to mischief or cause a reaction. Seed oils due to their unsaturated nature can cause an inflammatory reaction and frequently do.

You can see that animal fat has superior qualities when it comes to keeping the immune system well- balanced. Further, it contains some valuable vitamins which you will not find in seed oils and which we are often deficient in. For example, lard and full fat dairy milk contain very useful amounts of vitamin D. There are 4 fat soluble vitamins ADEK without which we would be ill very quickly given the diversity of their impact on the human body.

Of course our concern is that fat is also required for the active form of T3 to enter cells in order to function so when did low fat diets begin?

Around 1979, the American Society of Clinical Nutritionists, the National Cancer Institute and the AHA had all recommended low fat diets as healthy diets and this was further supported in 1980 when a scientific consensus began gathering support for this ideology especially in relation to cancers and coronary heart disease which were the two leading causes of death at the time.

The erroneous assumption that fat is responsible for much ill health has permeated society so much now that it will not be lifted easily, if ever.

Professor John Yudkin, author of Pure, White and Deadly, (1972 and 1986) identified the cause of ill health and it was not fat or cholesterol but refined sugar. However, his voice was drowned out by others even though his views were supported by many more concerned scientists.

Low fat diets were not just gaining popularity in the 1970's though. Keys, in the 1950's, promoted such a diet with an emphasis on less meat, more fruit and vegetables and olive oil to replace the animal fat

Without any real evidence the American Heart Association stated that reducing dietary fat intake would be followed by a reduced incidence of coronary heart disease. In 1961, this proposal was modified a little. A report[3] stated

'it must be emphasised that there is as yet no *final proof that heart attacks and strokes will be prevented by such measures.'*

Indeed, further clarification confirmed that the recommendations would only apply to a small section – those who had prior heart attack or stroke or some hereditary predisposition.

If further proof were needed, then we only have to look at the Atkins Diet where those participating in this novel way of eating – which

---

[3] https://academic.oup.com/jhmas/article/63/2/139/772615

involved large quantities of fat and modest amounts of protein - lost weight and lowered their blood pressure and blood sugars.

In the light of the success of the Atkins diet, the advice that people adopt a low fat diet was ill-advised but the AHA did state that a low fat diet was not suitable for everyone although it may have some use for those who had hereditary cardiovascular disease or previous history but even this did not have evidence to back it.

Part of what informed this advice was that fat contained more calories than either protein or carbohydrate, gram for gram and therefore may contribute to obesity. Fat does contain 9 calories per gram whilst carbohydrate and protein contain only 4. However, fat is the least likely to raise insulin levels and insulin levels really do matter when it comes to fat storage. In this respect fat is a clear winner when it comes to keep body mass down.

Weight never has been about 'more calories in than needed will put weight on.' The body is much more complex than that.

The moral of this story is that the thyroid machinery needs fat in order to run smoothly and it should not be cut out of the diet at any point including when there is a thyroid condition.

Selenium Deficiency in thyroid dysfunction and the relationship with viral pathogenesis

The world appears to be waking up to the fact that providing the immune system with adequate nutrition, including vitamin D and zinc, would offer protection against viruses in a way that man- made responses cannot. The lethality of our immune system is remarkably demonstrated in the cytokine storm. This occurs when immune system cells, get out of control and pour toxic chemicals on infected host cells in a bid to completely eradicate any viral presence.   An adequate intake of vitamin D is required to modulate any over activity by the immune system as well as synthesise antimicrobials known as cathelicidins that have particular efficacy against respiratory infections. In this we also have to consider whether our intake of magnesium is sufficient given that vitamin D cannot be activated without magnesium.

However, we must also consider selenium, another trace mineral which has well documented efficacy against viral pathogenesis. Selenium deficiency is not uncommon due to selenium deficient soils that many of our foodstuffs are grown in. However, as selenium is vital for the health of the immune system – both innate and adaptive immune systems - we cannot ignore the impact of any deficiency of this essential micronutrient for immune responses, thyroid health and oxidative damage prevention. Experimental animal studies show that there is a less robust immune response to viruses, tumours and allergies in those who are selenium deficient compared to controls.

Indeed, a publication from 2011[4] has argued that many virulent strains of enveloped viruses including SARS, Bird Flu and Ebola have spread to areas where selenium deficient soil is present.

Selenium replaces a sulphur atom in the amino acid cysteine which will ultimately become incorporated into selenoproteins. There are many selenoproteins of which glutathione peroxidase is the most well-known. Glutathione Peroxidase, in addition to other selenoproteins, slows down viral replication and mutation, reducing viral symptoms and infection times.

Selenium has particular efficacy against RNA enveloped viruses[5]. These include the polio virus, influenza A, HIV-1, enterovirus and many others. Covid 19 is also an RNA enveloped virus. Benign viruses are known to become

---

[4] https://link.springer.com/article/10.1007/s12011-011-8977-1
[5] Hori K, Hatfield D, Maldarelli F, Lee BJ, Clouse KA. Selenium supplementation suppresses tumor necrosis factor alpha-induced human immunodeficiency virus type 1 replication in vitro. AIDS Res Hum Retroviruses.

especially virulent in the presence of selenium deficiency.[6] Studies of selenium deficiency and Keshan disease – a condition prevalent in a particular area of China that has particularly selenium deficient soils, - show that supplementation of selenium to individuals with this disease completely prevents the development of this cardiomyopathic disease. The aetiology of Keshan disease is inextricably interwound with endemic Cocksackievirus. When selenium deficiency is corrected, antiviral immunity is enhanced and RNA mutation into a more severe form of virus is prevented. The condition resolves.

The concept of preventing virus from mutating into more severe strains – whether by drift or shift – is an important one if we are to avoid further waves of viral infection that may see individuals with only partial or no protection to a new wave. Lockdown should not be the answer not only because of the damage to the economy but it disadvantages many of those in

---

[6] https://www.ncbi.nlm.nih.gov/pubmed/8083665/

society who are not offered treatment for other medical conditions.

Thyroid dysfunction can also disrupt many other functions in the body. For example, it is associated with hypo-motility of the gastro intestinal tract leading to constipation. However, it may also promote bacterial overgrowth resulting in small intestinal bacterial overgrowth (SIBO) and this may result in chronic diarrhoea.

West German scientists have found that selenium is an essential component of an enzyme in the thyroid gland. Selenium is part of the enzyme deiodinase which catalyses the production of trilothyronin (T3) from thyroxine (T4). In cases where there is a selenium deficiency, there will not be enough of the enzyme present.

Selenium deficiency is rare in well-nourished individuals but poor diets, malabsorption problems and ageing, where nutrients are generally poorly absorbed, anyway, are some of the most at risk groups. Two Brazil nuts provide all your daily selenium requirements. Other good sources are mainly of animal origin and include, liver, seafood eggs, milk, yogurt, muscle meats, fortified grains and cereals.

NSAID's and their impact on thyroxine levels

Apart from carrageen, many other substances impact the ability of the thyroid to function correctly.

A study sought to investigate the effects of nonsteroidal anti-inflammatory drugs (NSAIDs) on thyroid tests. This involved 25 healthy subjects subject to a single dose study or a 1-week study.

The single dose study involved subjects receiving a single dose of either:

Aspirin

Salsalate

Meclofenamate

Ibuprofen

Naproxen

Indomethacin

Total and free thyroid hormones were analysed as was TSH at the hours of

0,1,2,3, and 8 hours

The one-week study[7] involved participants being given one of the 6 NSAIDs for 7 days and analysis of the TSH and thyroid hormones were analysed at 0800.

---

[7] https://pubmed.ncbi.nlm.nih.gov/14671157/

No changes were detected in any of the hormones after a single dose or after one week of ibuprofen, indomethacin or naproxen.

However, the single dose aspirin and the salsalate decreased the hormones whilst the meclofenamate increased the hormones.

A one-week total aspirin decreased total T4 but the free T4 was seen to decrease in the salsalate only.

Total T3, free T3 and TSH were found to decrease in both the aspirin and salsalate while there was an increase in the Meclofenamate across all.

If this were tabulated for ease of access it would appear like this overleaf:

Table showing the action of common NSAID's on the thyroid hormones after one week.

NSAID	Impact on T3	Impact on T4	Impact on TSH
Aspirin	decrease	decrease	decrease
Salsalate	decrease	Decrease (free T4 only)	decrease
Meclofenamate	increase	increase	Increase
Ibuprofen	No change	No change	No change
Naproxen	No change	No change	No change
Indomethacin	No change	No change	No change

It should be noted that the TSH remained within the normal range during acute or one-week administration of the NSAID's. However, the impact of Salsalate and Aspirin may add to the cumulative effects of other products which affect good thyroid function as well as causing more severe inhibition of thyroid functioning over a longer time scale.

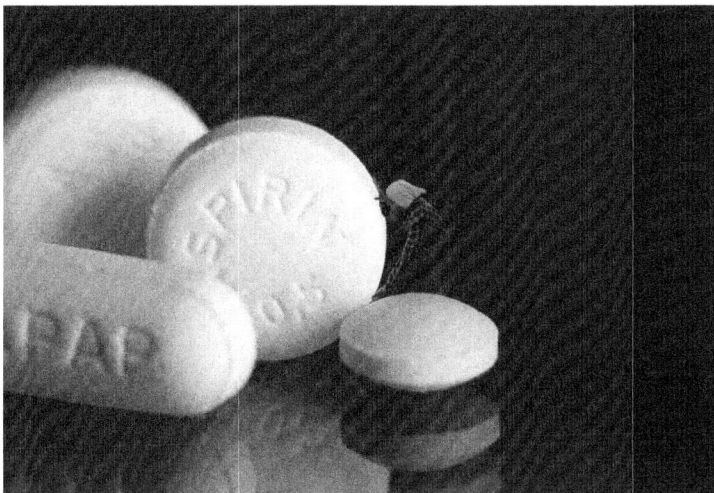

Aspirin inhibits T3 and T4

Goitregens

Goitregens are one class of many classes of ant nutrients which exist in the plant world. Anti-nutrients are the defensive traits found in a plant which prevent them from being eaten. Unfortunately, they not only make some plants unpalatable to some herbivores but they do have the potential to inhibit essential trace minerals necessary for the optimum working of the thyroid gland – including iodine and zinc – from being absorbed. We then say they are not bioavailable.

We are probably more used to hearing about the anti-nutrient phytic acid in relation to its inhibition of zinc -which it binds to avidly - thus rendering it non-bioavailable. Zinc, of course, is also vital for thyroid function. However, goitregens are anti-nutrients which specifically interfere with how the body can use iodine.

The two main sources of goitregens are:

Soy products

Cruciferous vegetables

Cruciferous vegetables belong to the Brassicaceae family and these include:

Cauliflower, kale, turnips and Brussels sprouts which contain good amounts of an indole known as glucosinolate.

An indole is an aromatic organic compound widely distributed in the environment. It has been found, in animal studies, to be degraded into a goitrin metabolite.

A metabolite is a small molecule used in metabolism or is the end product of metabolism.

In this case the goitrin metabolite is called thiocyanate. Thiocyanate inhibits iodine uptake by the cells found in the thyroid. As such the synthesis of thyroid hormones is disrupted.

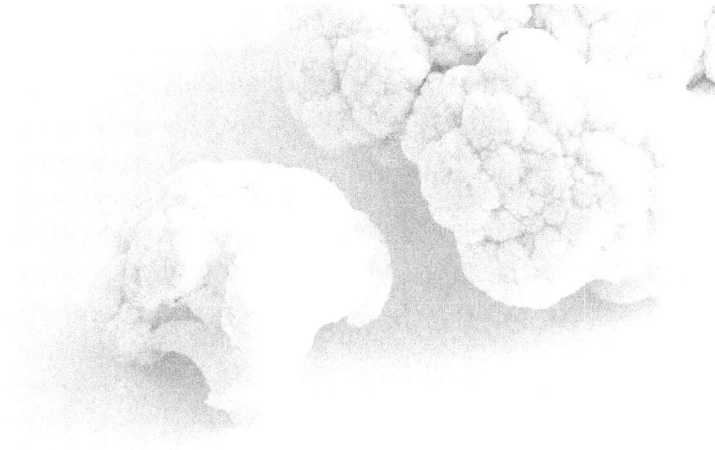

Cauliflower can disrupt the synthesis of thyroid hormone

How much of these thyroid hormone disrupting plants can we eat before they impact the thyroid?

This is one of those, 'how long is a piece of string questions?' In some people it may mean very little. Others may have to consume much larger quantities but what is fairly certain is that a plant based diet may be detrimental to those who consume it.

Data on this particular subject is limited. However, there has been a small study carried out on 5 healthy subjects which showed a decrease of approximately 25% of the uptake of radioiodine after consumption of kale juice twice daily for a period of one week. The thyroid function tests, however, remained unchanged.

Other studies have shown that consuming large amounts of pak choi was associated with myxoedema. The amount of pak choi was excessive – in the region of just over 1kg daily for an extended period but, nevertheless, evidences the impact of goitregens on thyroid function.

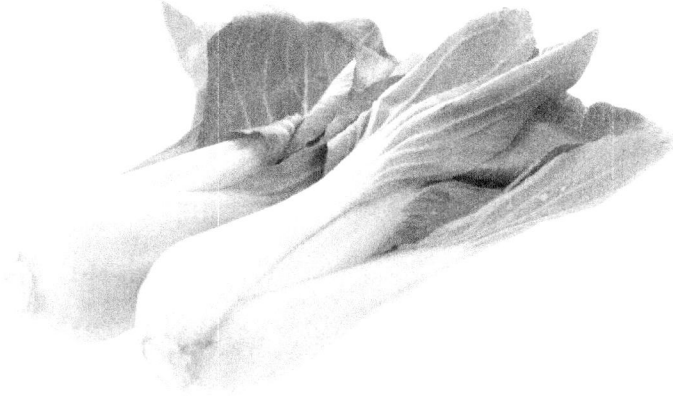

Eating quantities of pak choi is not helpful for those with thyroid problems as it impacts thyroid hormones, negatively.

Cooking food does destroy the goitrogenic metabolite but then so many vitamins are lost too in the process. Further, many of the trace elements which are vital for thyroid function leach into the cooking water which most people throw away.

In addition, soy products contain goitregens. Soy products are big news at the moment. Consumers are encouraged to drink soya milk (to save the planet), eat soy based yogurts, textured vegetable protein and use soy flour. Soy is added to most ready meals including tinned soups. It is hard to avoid.

The isoflavone in soy inhibits thyroid hormones in those with iodine deficiency.

A case report[8] from the 1960's found that a baby on a soybean formula for 4 months developed a goitre which began to correct itself within a week of removing the soy milk and replacing it with dairy.

Further pearl millet grain has also been found to cause goitre   by suppressing the function of the thyroid gland. This is better understood in the light of those living in rural parts of Asia and Africa where millet grain is their staple diet. In these areas, goitre is endemic.

---

[8] https://www.ncbi.nlm.nih.gov/pmc/articles/PMC7282437/#B17

How does pearl millet grain impact the thyroid? Well, it is rich in something called C-glycosylflavones which has been found in studies to inhibit 85% of the thyroid peroxidase enzyme. This enzyme has a major role to play in the production of thyroid hormones.

It is found in the thyroid.

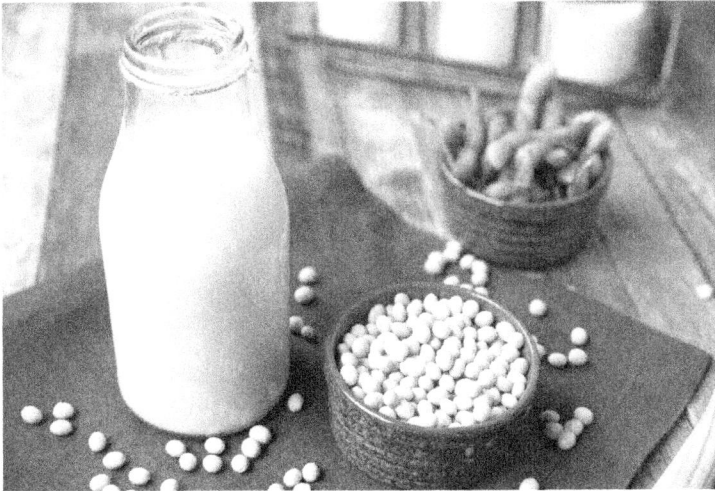

Soy milk is not thyroid friendly.

peanut oil is also a potential goitregens and was consumed in large quantities in the post WW2 era.

Moreover, onions and garlic have been found to have potential goitregens[9]

It seems that our 'healthy' plant based diets are not so healthy after all – at least not for those with a vulnerability to thyroid problems.

As we have seen the impact of anti-nutrients on thyroid function, we should also look at how supplements can impact the absorption of medications prescribed for the thyroid.

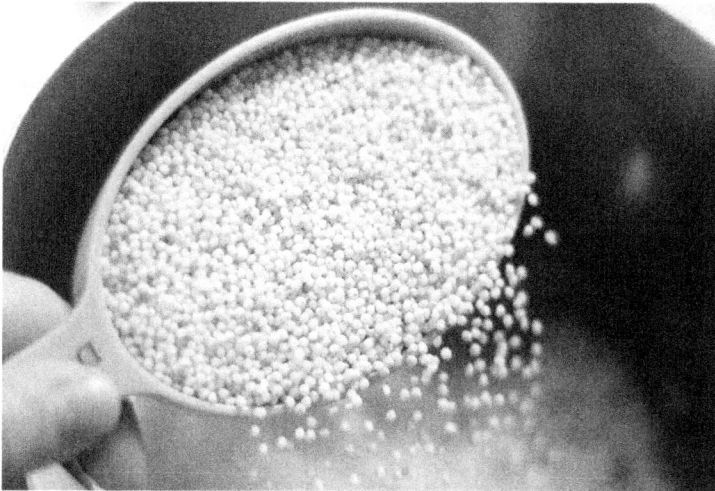

9 https://www.ncbi.nlm.nih.gov/pmc/articles/PMC7282437/#B23

Millet grain is often eaten by vegetarians as an additional grain to the more popular ones like oats. Unfortunately, it is not thyroid friendly.

Supplements and thyroid function

Many supplements impact thyroid function. Unfortunately, they are ones that are commonly given out or recommended. For example, calcium is regularly given to the elderly to try and reduce the progression of osteoporosis although there could be many reasons why this condition has manifested itself and few, are to do with the amount of calcium that has been ingested.

Calcium is known to interfere with thyroid medications but I have not known anyone yet who has been informed of this by their doctor. Coffee and fibre – yes that fibre that has been pushed onto us as being healthy – will also inhibit the absorption of thyroid medication.

The nutrient, chromium picolinate, is well known as a nutrient which helps to lower blood sugar. It is often used by diabetics as an alternative treatment to Metformin and other treatments frequently prescribed for diabetics.

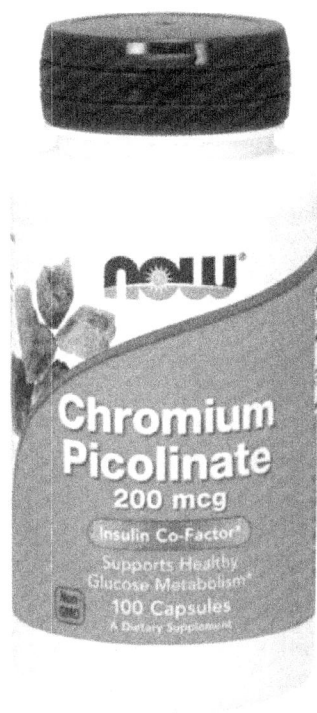

It is also used for weight loss. However, it does inhibit the absorption of thyroid medications.

As with all supplements, medications or food items which have the potential to impair thyroid medication it is by far the better to take the medication well before any of the offending items, giving it chance to be absorbed first.

Let's look at chromium a little further.

Chromium exists in many forms but only the trivalent chromium can be used in the body. It is an essential trace element for us.

Chromium has one main function which is known as Glucose Tolerance Factor (GTF).

GTF stimulates insulin activity by binding to insulin and the specific insulin receptors. Therefore, GTF:

Suppresses hunger symptoms through the brain satiety centre

Stimulates the production of essential nerve substances

Increases resistance to infection

Controls blood glucose by enabling its uptake by muscles and organs as well as increasing the ability of glucose to be used for energy.

Helps control blood glucose levels

Reduces arteriosclerosis

Stimulates protein synthesis

Controls blood cholesterol levels

So, as you can see, it has a wide range of functions.

Absorption from food is very poor and a good amount is lost through faeces and urine daily.

The best food sources of chromium are:

Egg yolk

Wheat germ

Cereals

Honey

Bran

Hard cheese

Beef

Dried brewer's yeast

Molasses

Liver – whether pigs, lambs or beef liver

Fruit and vegetables also contain some but you may wish to reduce your intake if you are looking to improve your thyroid function.

Highly refined diets and food refining and processing are not advisable as most of the chromium will have been removed.

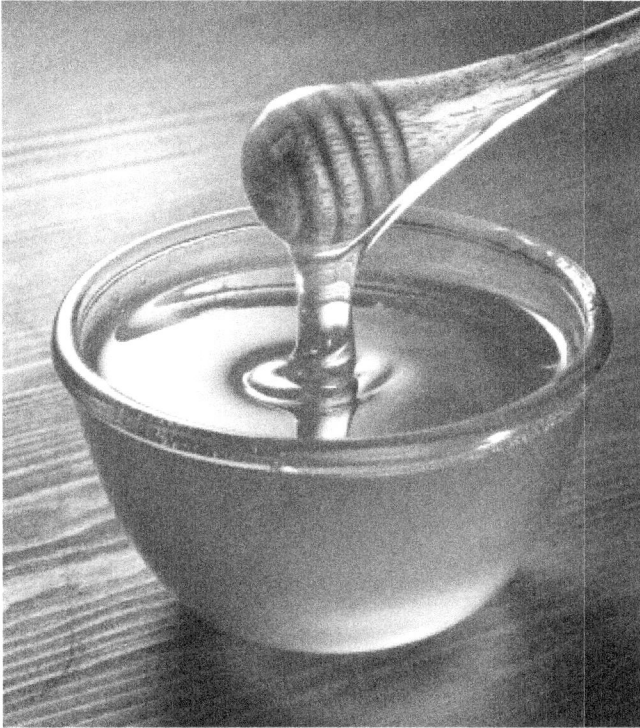

Honey contains chromium in useful amounts

Yeast is probably the best supplement for chromium as it contains the chromium as GTF which is 50 times more effective than other forms of chromium and is 20 times more readily absorbed.

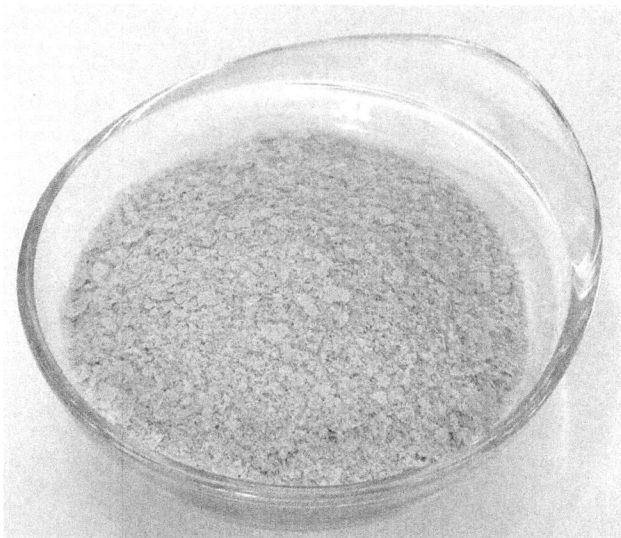

Nutritional yeast flakes are a popular addition to soups and stews and provide good amounts of chromium.

It should also be noted that the incidence of diabetes and heart disease does decrease with increasing levels of chromium in the diet. One very good reason why pubs contribute to health apart from supporting the social aspect necessary for mental health.

So after this minor, but useful diversion, into the benefits of chromium, it can be seen that, while in some ways, it can be very beneficial for some, those with a propensity to thyroid dysfunction may not fare so well.   However, I would say that some people with a thyroid disorder may also have a propensity to prediabetes or diabetes and it may be in this case that chromium may help and the thyroid patient may well consider looking elsewhere for the cause of their dysfunctional thyroid other than an excess of chromium in their diet. We must never lose sight of the multiplicity of ways that thyroid activity can be affected.

So now, it is time to look at further causes of suppressed thyroid function.

Unfortunately, flavonoids in tea, fruit and vegetables have the potential to suppress thyroid function.

What are flavonoids?

These are compounds which occur naturally in fruits, vegetables, tea, coffee and wine.

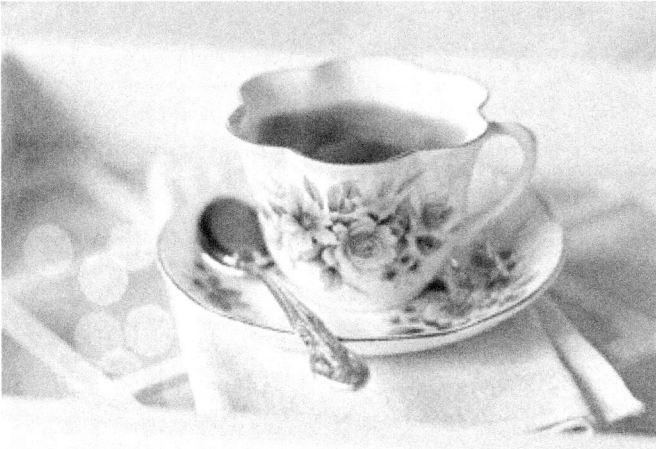

Excessive tea drinking is not beneficial to thyroid function

There are six classes of flavonoids found in food. Each one is metabolised differently in the body.

Flavonoids have their uses. They can reduce inflammatory activity and neutralise toxins. However, antioxidants in animal products tend to have far greater impact than flavonoids. Further, plant based foods contain the sugar

71

fructose which can have further detrimental impact on the body.

Let's have a look at the different types of Flavanoids.

Flavanols

Generally known for their beneficial impact on cardiovascular disease, they are found in:

Peaches, berries, tea, coffee, onions, kale, grapes, red wine, broccoli, tomatoes and lettuce

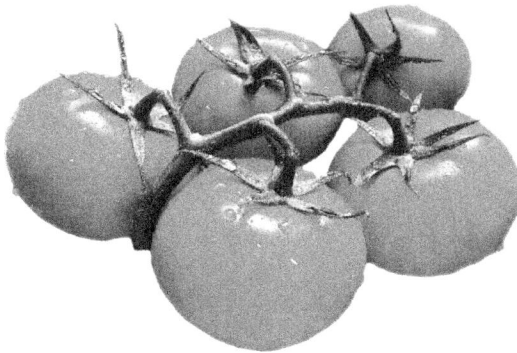

Eating tomatoes and tomato based products excessively, may contribute to thyroid dysfunction.

Flavan-3-ols

These are found in all types of tea, green, black and white, apples, red or purple grapes, blueberries, strawberries, cocoa and products containing them.

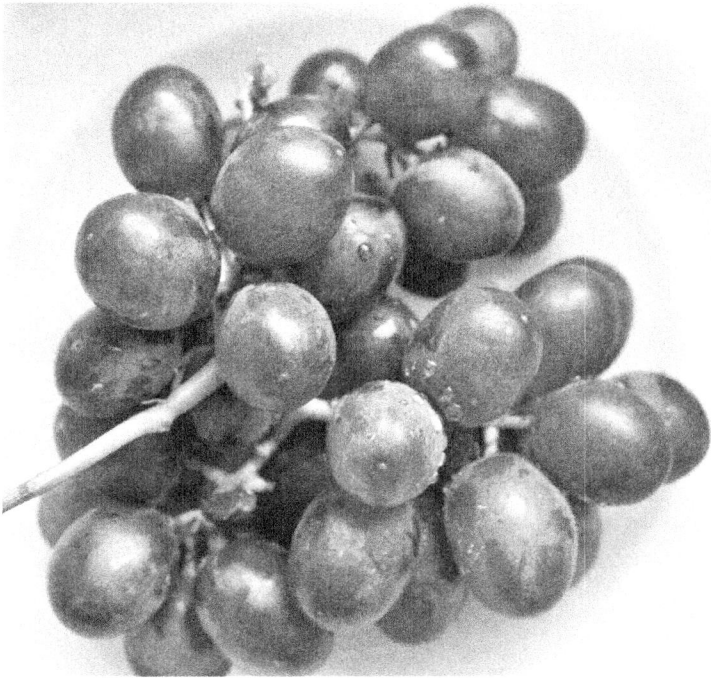

Red grapes may impact thyroid function negatively if eaten in excessive amounts or with other flavonoids.

Flavanones

Generally known for their anti-inflammatory properties, they are found in citrus fruit.

Flavones

These are found in blue and white coloured plants and are a natural insecticide which helps protect the plant from attack. They are normally found in red peppers, celery, parsley, peppermint and chamomile. The supplement apigenin normally contains large amounts of this flavone.

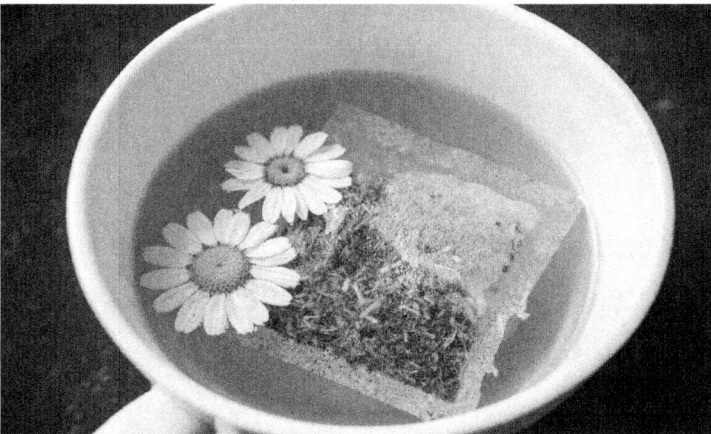

Chamomile tea, a favourite of healthy food addicts, can inhibit the normal workings of the thyroid.

Isoflavones

Isoflavonoids are found mainly in soy products which have crept into many of our ready meals now including soups. They are also found in legumes with fava bean, which contain some L-dopa, the precursor of the neurotransmitter, dopamine, containing the highest amounts.

Anthocyanins

Cyan, of course, relates to the colour blue so you will find these in in plants which are pigmented with blue, purple or red tones.

Thus, the majority of berries will contain anthocyanins as would red wine, cranberries, blackberries, elderberries among many others.

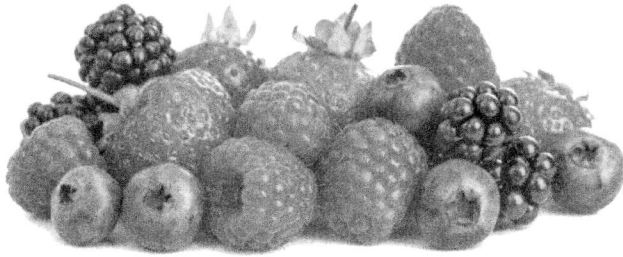

Berries eaten in excessive quantities may disrupt thyroid function

Although many sources state that flavonoids are beneficial, there are equally as many sources which do not agree with this. With respect to thyroid function, it appears that a diet overly rich in flavonoids is not beneficial and a something along the lines of a keto diet may be more appropriate.

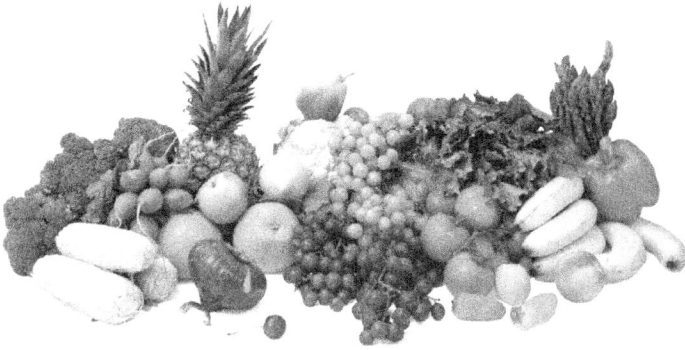

Fruit and vegetables are not as healthy optimum thyroid function as we have been led to believe.

In a keto diet, small amounts of fruit and vegetables may be eaten but these are unlikely to be in the quantities that would disrupt the workings of the thyroid.

The Amino Acid Tyrosine

It should be fairly obvious now that there is not one single trace mineral or vitamin that works in isolation from many others. The way the body systems work are exquisitely choreographed and the exclusion or deficiency of one or more of them will cause some form of syndrome or condition to arise. This is why the mantra regarding a balanced diet needs to be repeated over and over again. Therapeutic tweaks such as including supplemental vitamin D are the exception and not the rule.

Will we ever get back to eating without the numerous food fads inflicted on society by those celebrities whose unusual diets habits are followed slavishly by those wishing to contribute to the profits of their numerous books.

No one has yet written a book on the post WW2 diet which was admirable since all resources were employed in the diet to produce a well-rounded and nutritious diet to produce healthy children to replace the millions that died during that war.

Tyrosine is an important amino acid when it comes to thyroxine for iodine needs to combine with the amino acid tyrosine in order to form thyroxine. Thyroxine simply cannot be synthesised without both of these substances in the right proportions for any specific individual.

Sadly, far too much has been written about vitamins and minerals to the detriment of knowledge of the necessity for amino acids. A paucity of specific amino acids is rarely mentioned as a cause of a condition. However, once you start taking food groups out then it is quite likely that certain amino acids will not be found in the required quantities. We may find, if we search hard enough, that certain conditions appear to be rifer in certain fad diets.

We do know that iron deficiency anaemia is rifer in vegan diets as would be a vitamin D deficiency with the knock on effect on bone and immune system health that such a deficiency could lead to. Vegan diets are also deficient in vitamin B12 which is very much associated with dementia like symptoms.

When thyroid problems are present, most people will reach for the iodine supplements (with the risk of causing the thyroid to go into meltdown trying to keep up with the onslaught) but never have I heard from patient or medic alike that attention to the tyrosine intake in their diet must be made. Such is life.

In good health, the body has an amazing capacity to address the problems of sub and malnutrition. It simply breaks down some tissues in the body somewhere and 'borrows' what it needs. As the body ages, this avenue is not open to it as freely as it was and the inaccessibility of vital nutrients simply leads to disease. The thyroid is no different. Rarely do we ever see thyroid dysfunction in children on the scale we see in the over 50's.

The precursor of tyrosine is phenylalanine – that amino acid that tends to end up in energy drinks. Phenylalanine is the parent substance of dopamine, norepinephrine (noradrenaline) and epinephrine (adrenaline) for which vitamins B6 and C are essential in the conversion process.

The whole process is much more complex than I can give in a book like this, other nutrient deficiencies will also impact this process negatively but the above shows how easy it is for a condition to occur as a simple nutrient deficiency.

Phenylalanine has many roles besides the one involved in its conversion to tyrosine and these may give clues as to whether you are deficient in it.

These include:

Depression

Pain

Vitiligo – the depigmentation in the skin

Cognitive deficits

Inability to form a sun tan with reasonable amounts of sunlight exposure.

Tyrosine, which is derived from phenylalanine, is a precursor of dopa, dopamine, norepinephrine and adrenaline.

Strangely, adequate amounts of tyrosine have been found to be effective in alleviating hay fever and grass allergies. It is therefore likely that those suffering similar allergies may not only have a vulnerability to thyroid disorders but may also be susceptible to Parkinson's disease and similar.

This is an important point because Parkinson's like symptoms rarely occur before 80% of the area of the brain affected by Parkinson's disease (substantia nigra) has already been damaged. Being able to relate other conditions which may point to the possibility of such a degenerative condition, may mean we can do something about it before any potential condition is advanced and hence, less amenable to reversal.

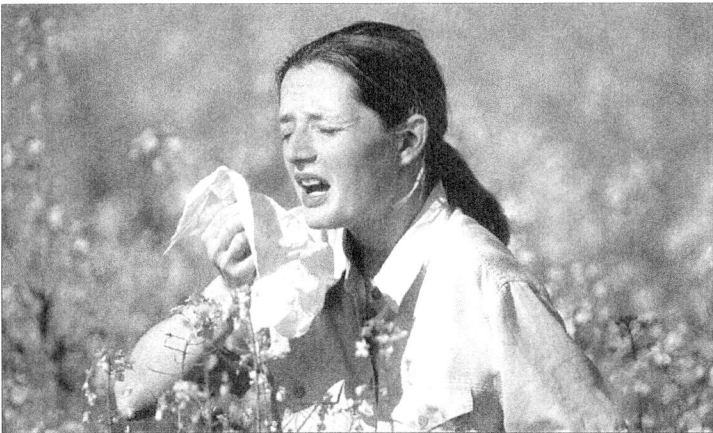

Hay fever type allergies are linked to thyroid dysfunction.

Phenylalanine gives rise to many other symptoms which include – but are not confined to:

Blood shot eyes

Cataracts

Behavioural changes

Lack of appetite control - taken at doses of 100mg-500mg before a retiring would suppress appetite for the following day. However, if overall protein intake is low and this single amino acid is taken then it could induce a tyrosine toxicity which could result in depression and eye lesions.

Some of the deficiency symptoms of tyrosine deficiency include:

Low blood pressure

Restless legs

Low body temperature

Lack of skin and hair pigmentation

Tyrosine is capable of producing toxic reaction in excessive doses or if phenylalanine intake is excessive.

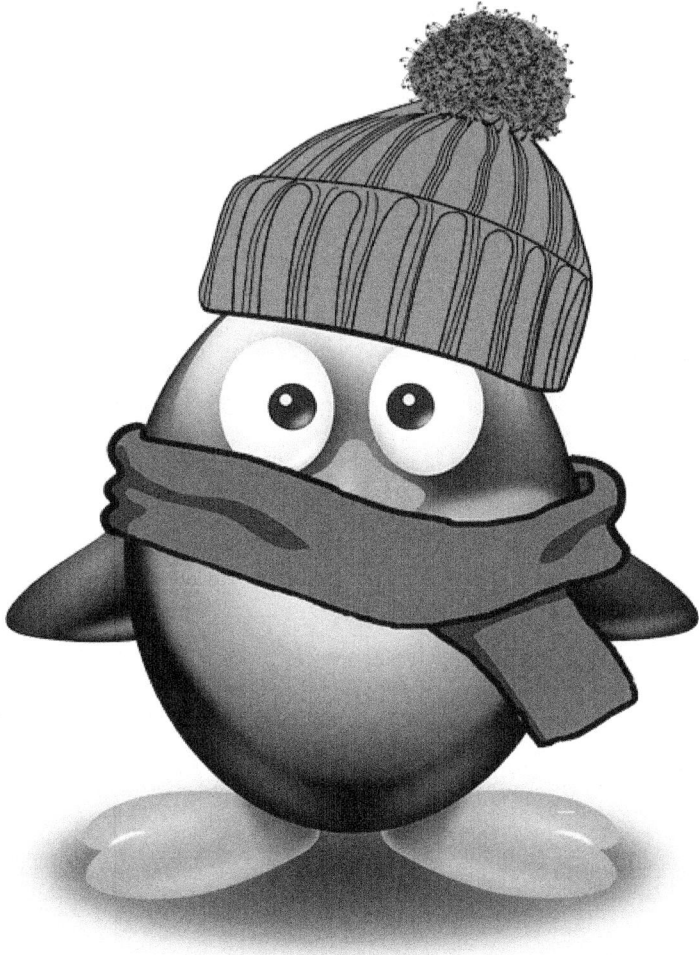

Feeling cold is a sign of tyrosine deficiency

The sources of phenylalanine are animal derived and include:

Eggs, poultry, organ meats, red meat and white meat, seafoods like salmon, trout and tuna, lobster and shrimp.

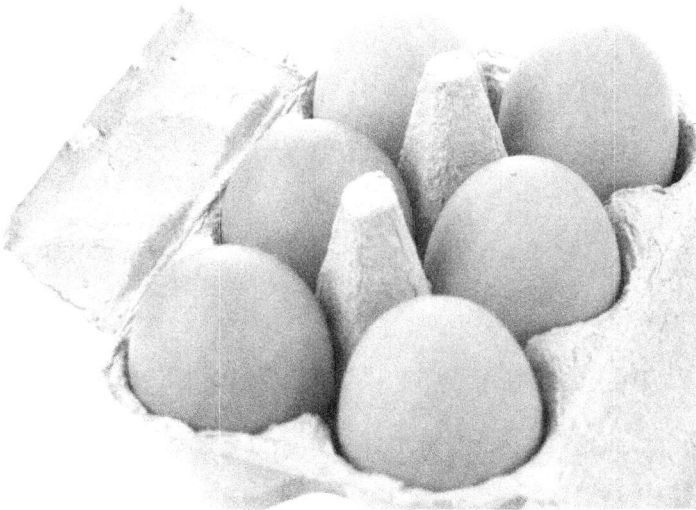

Eggs are a good source of phenylalanine

Plant sources of phenylalanine include:

Nuts of all varieties, seeds, nut butters such as peanut butter and legumes such as kidney beans.

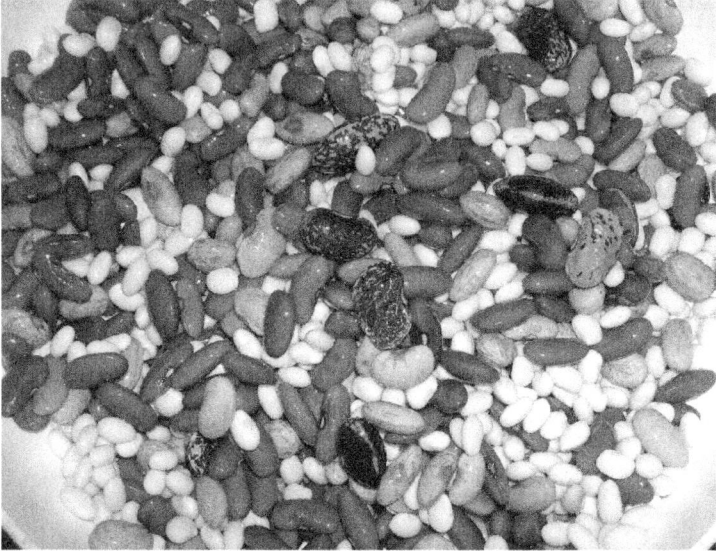

Beans of all types contain phenylalanine

The sources of tyrosine are more or less the same provided you take into account the conversion of such which requires vitamin B6 and vitamin C to aid that conversion.

Therefore, good sources of vitamin B6 – Pyroxidone- which should be taken in conjunction with the B complex as a whole include:

Dried brewer's yeast

Wheat bran

Yeast extract

Oat flakes

Eggs

Vegetables

Potatoes

Brown rice

Pig's liver

Oily fish

Meat

Nuts

Bananas

Soya flour

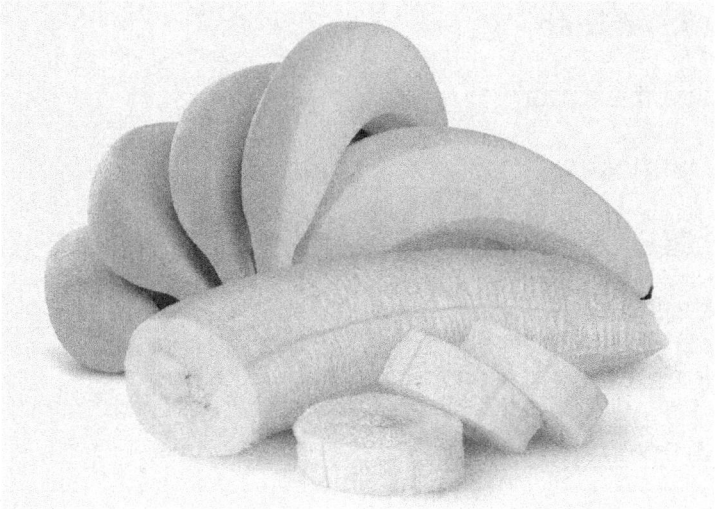

bananas are a good source of vitamin B6

Pyroxidone is easily destroyed in heated milk and deficiency symptoms which may occur are:

Lips splitting

Inflamed tongue

Puffy ankles and fingers

Swollen abdomen

Breast discomfort

Irritability

Migraine

Inflamed nerve endings

Mild depression

Scaly skin on face

Deficiency can be caused by a number of reasons including:

Contraceptive pill

Many drugs including penicillamine

Alcohol and smoking

Some dependency states are asthma, urticaria, mental retardation, premenstrual tension, kidney stones and atherosclerosis where higher doses of pyroxidone are called for.

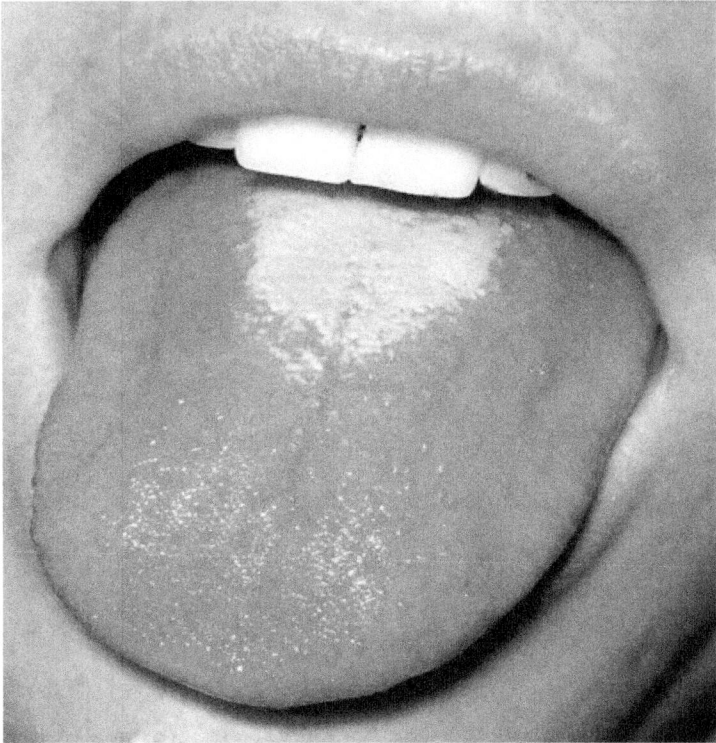

An inflamed tongue is a sign of pyroxidone deficiency

Most people know the sources of vitamin C. Collecting rose hips post war to make rose hip syrup was part and parcel of that era to make sure that people had enough of this vital nutrient in their diet.

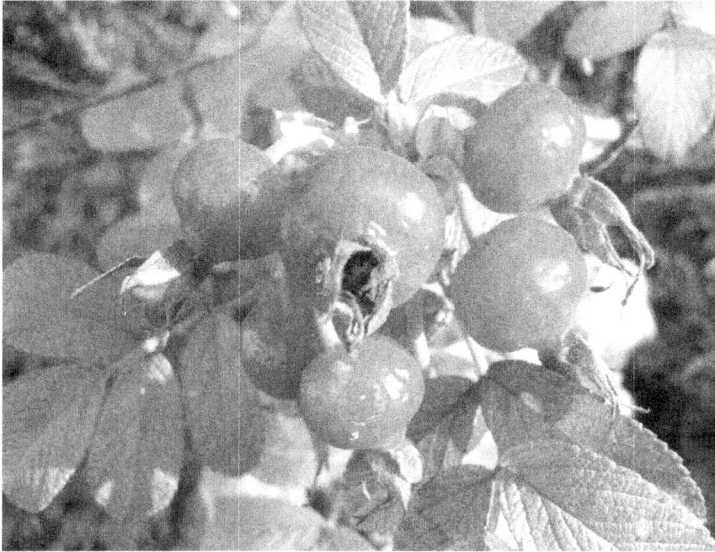

People used to gather rose hips post war to make into some syrup rich in vitamin C

Most people think that only fruit and veg contain vitamin C but, of course, meat does. Vitamin C is a co-factor in many bodily processes including those found in muscle.

Vitamin C has many functions apart from its role in the synthesis of thyroxine from iodine and tyrosine.   For example, it is an antioxidant, promotes iron absorption, produces the anti-stress hormone, helps resist infection, controls blood cholesterol levels and helps the maintenance of healthy collagen. People with young looking skins tend to have a diet well supplied with vitamin C. It is also required to activate folic acid.

There's that interdependence on other nutrients.

Further, vitamin C helps maintain healthy bones, healthy teeth, a healthy blood system, sex organs and is well known as nature's anti-histamine

Vitamin C is quite an unstable vitamin being easily destroyed by heat and light such that when milk was delivered to the door, housewives were told to take it in immediately so that the sunlight would not degrade the vitamin.

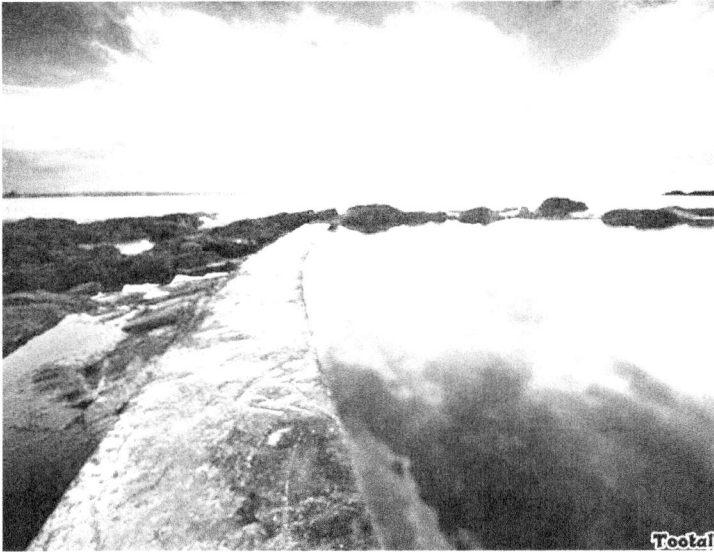

Sunlight degrades vitamin C rapidly.

In clear deficiency of vitamin C, it is manifested as scurvy and there are some people who need to take more of this nutrient if they are to avoid a deficiency. These include those who take:

Aspirin

Contraceptive pill

Antibiotics

Barbiturates

Corticosteroids

Anti-arthritic drugs

Those enduring stressful events

The elderly

Athletes

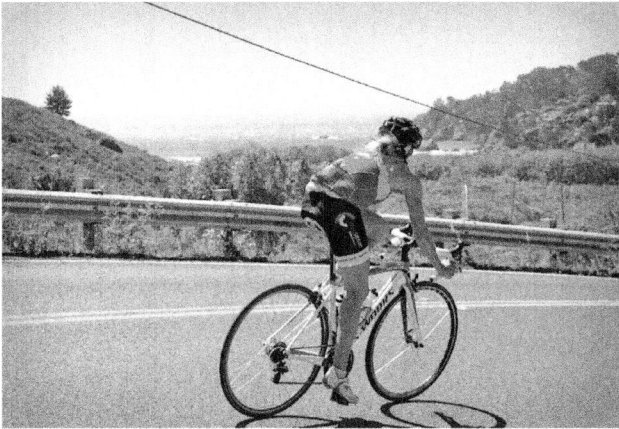

Athletes need extra vitamin C in order to avoid deficiency symptoms

Those undergoing dental surgery or indeed any form of surgery.

Those with an infection

Those with an injury

Diabetics

Alcohol

Those with gastric and duodenal ulcers

Clear deficiency symptoms include:

Weakness

Easy bruising or haemorrhages in the skin, eyes and nose

Gingivitis and loosening of the teeth

Bleeding gums

Fatigue and a 'can't be bothered' feeling

Muscle and joint pains

irritability

Surprisingly, the best sources are not citrus fruit as we have been led to believe but Brussels sprouts which provides 90mg per 100g. However, you have to consider that Brussels sprouts are a major goitregens. Yes, cooking will degrade the goitregens but it will also degrade the vitamin C that is contained within them. Who thought nutrition could be so complex?

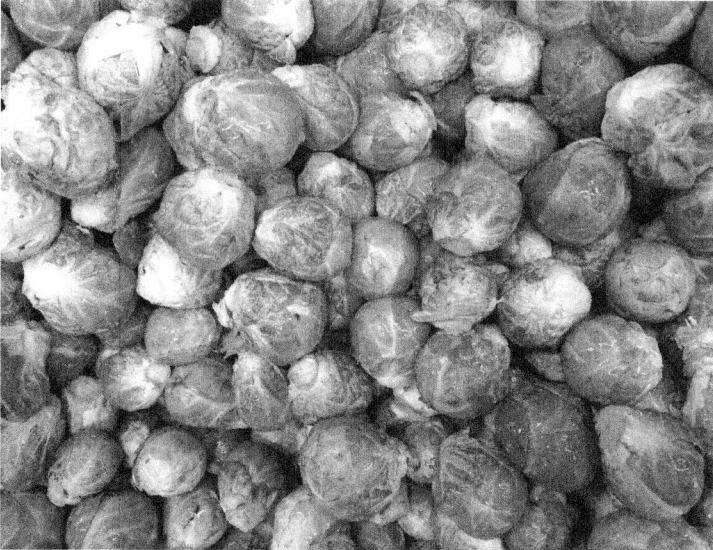

Sprouts contain good amounts of vitamin C but also contain goitregens. They are the thyroid patient's dilemma.

Other sources of vitamin C are:

Citrus fruits

Watercress

Cabbage

Mustard tops

Other fruit and vegetables

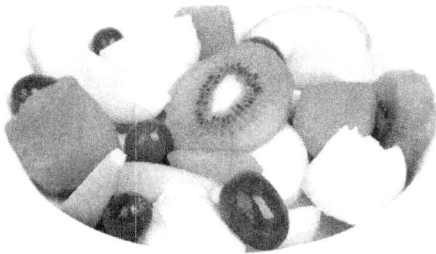

A dishful of vitamin C as long as it is very fresh and eaten straight away

Vitamin C is generally considered to be a safe vitamin but excessive intake can cause symptoms of:

Nausea

Abdominal cramps

Diarrhoea

But this is unlikely if the dosage remains under 3g daily.

I have included the symptoms of excessive intake of vitamin C because it is a vitamin that is very much supplemented to excess nowadays and one of the side effects of diarrhoea is the loss of vitamin B complex and zinc, among others which are necessary for the health of the thyroid.

Whenever any condition exists it is good to become acquainted with the deficiency symptoms of the nutrients that are needed for the optimal function of that organ or system. Being aware can alert you to rectifying the problem before it creates further problems. The need for increasing thyroxine does not bode well for those with a family vulnerability to Parkinson's disease.   The return of an urticarial like condition or hay fever could alert you to the fact that the thyroid is struggling. As vitamin C adequately addresses these conditions could it be that a vitamin C deficiency is causing the need for more thyroxine to be synthesised? It's not all about iodine but while GP's and patients are fixated upon it, they will not look beyond to see the wider complexity of this bodily system.

Before I leave the subject of vitamin C, I should add that for every cigarette that is smoked, 30mg of vitamin C will, on average, be used up.

Smokers generally tend to feel stress. It may be one of the reasons why they started smoking in the first place. Stress also uses vitamin C up rapidly.   The smoker's propensity to eat less because of the impact of smoking also means that they are likely to be suffering from malnutrition or sub nutrition.   Even from this fairly simple scenario it can be seen how one simple habit can lead to all sorts of conditions which do not appear to be related to others. This would also include thyroid dysfunction.

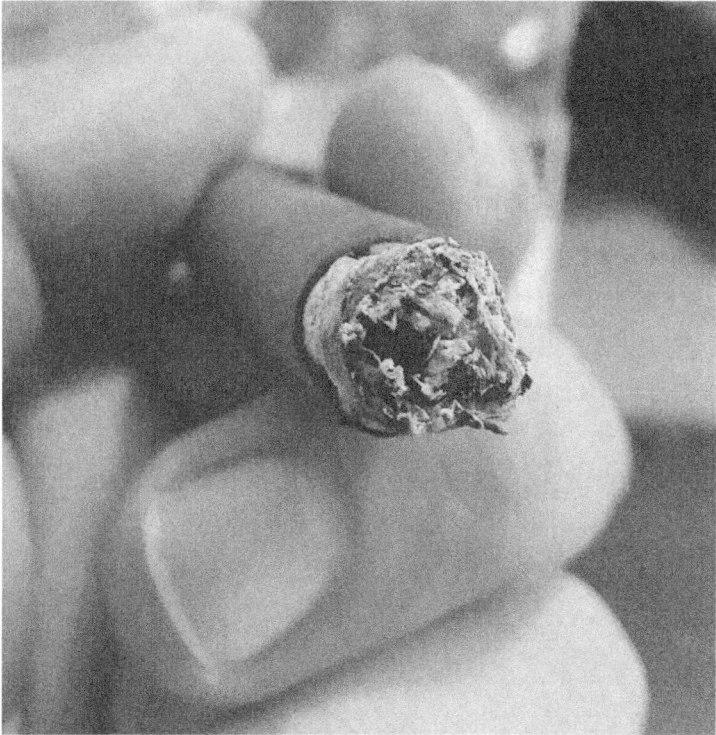

Smokers are at high risk of vitamin C deficiency and this will impact the thyroid in susceptible people.

The ageing process should not be of concern. Like any life stage it presents its joys and challenges and differential nutritional needs.

We understand these needs much more readily when we look at the transition of a baby to a pre- toddler. Most people can reel off why the nutritional needs should and must change i.e. breast milk does not contain iron and the baby will only have enough iron for 6 months. We understand that needs change when the child is a little older and that they will eat 'like a horse' when they are teenagers and will not put an ounce on. We know what expectant mothers need to eat prior to conception and during pregnancy but then it seems to stop at over 50's will need to take a vitamin D supplement along with calcium. Really, is that all!

There is no mention that appetite will reduce and in order to ingest the nutrients that are needed for health we are looking at smaller, maybe more frequent and nutritionally denser foods.

Those over 50 years are really not considered that much when it comes to their changing needs.

If these needs are not adapted to then chronic illness will follow just like the baby who was fed on soya milk and developed a goitre. Life stages have to be adapted to in order to avoid illness.

It has been mooted often that one of the reasons that chronic illness occurs in this age group is that absorption of nutrients is not as effective and I would concur with that. However, this may well be because of a lack of gastric acid which is required in order to break down food effectively so that it can be absorbed. Rectifying a simple vitamin B1 deficiency would correct that problem within a couple of days and it is so easy to become thiamine (vitamin B1) deficient.

Excessive coffee and tea drinking degrades thiamine

High carbohydrate diets use up thiamine rapidly

Alcohol degrades thiamine

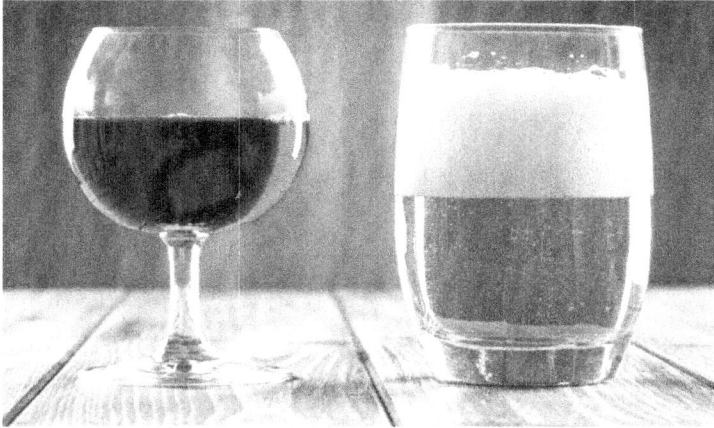

Many medications including Metformin, the diabetic medication, degrade thiamine.

What would be the likely response to a complaint of chronic aches and pains or similar?

'It's your age, you will have to learn to live with it'

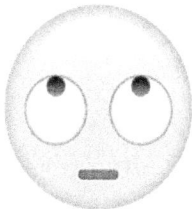

Older age should not be one of aches and pains and more chronic conditions than other life stages. Such symptoms tell us something is wrong and we need to investigate and address it.

I cannot think of anything more depressing than being told you have to live with a distressing and often painful condition for the rest of your life.

Other conditions related to thyroid dysfunction due to impaired nutritional pathways include but are not restricted to:

Vitiligo

Cataracts

Parkinson's disease

Depression

High cholesterol or unusual cholesterol levels

Atherosclerosis

Chronic immune gastritis

Sjogren disease

Rheumatoid arthritis

Multiple sclerosis

Polymyalgia rheumatica

Coeliac disease

Diabetes

Alopecia

Psoriatic arthritis

Addison's disease

Ulcerative colitis

You may want to find the common nutritional pathways which begin to bind these conditions together.

Other books by this author include:

- The EDS and Hypermobility Syndrome Diet
- Alleviating Symptoms of EDS
- Gastroparesis
- The EDS recipe book
- The Lipoedema Diet
- The Lymphoedema Diet: reverse and repair lymphatic damage
- The Anti-Virus Diet
- The Asthma Diet
- The Reluctant Bowel
- The MND Diet
- Why we live longer with higher cholesterol levels
- A dietary connection for MACS, POTS and EDS
- Identity: a self-exploration workbook *
- Journey Through Pneumonia

- Parkinson's Disease: dietary changes that work
- https://www.amazon.co.uk/dp/B07TBHMV6N

*This book can be used alone or in small group work and is an excellent resource for those who are 'people helpers.'

Among many others

They are available on Amazon

Lynne has written a semi-autobiographical trilogy.

For the full range of books by this author, visit the author website on

https://www.amazon.co.uk/-/e/B07BPQZ5CD

https://www.amazon.com/-/e/B07BPQZ5CD

A percentage of the profits from the sale of these books go to support charities like the Exodus Project below.

The Exodus Project

My first introduction to the far reaching impact of The Exodus Project occurred when I was travelling around Cawthorne in one of their buses, visiting gardens.   A young lad was happily munching on a sandwich. He looked up briefly, pointed to the driver and said,' He's my second dad, he is,' then he returned to his sandwich without further comment

Such remarks are often very telling and so I arranged to meet Jackie Peel and Martin Sawdon, at the charity's premises in Barnsley. They set up the Exodus Project 20 years ago. They moved into their current premises – a redundant Methodist church - in 2010.

Both Jackie and Martin have been youth workers in their church. Martin worked in housing for the homeless in addition to working in learning disabilities services in institutional settings.

The work that the Exodus Project undertakes is of paramount importance to the communities it serves. These were former mining communities which became disadvantaged after pit-closures. Currently about 400 children attend mid-week activities from Monday to Thursday inclusive. These activities include dance, drama, craft, music, sports and games. In addition, there are weekend camps, cycle treks, outward bound activities, bowling and swimming. The children are taught valuable life skills including how to cook and bake. It is all about teaching children how to fulfil their potential and learn skills they will be able to pass onto the next generation.

The grounds, once overgrown, have been turned into a play- and camping - ground. A miniature railway is in the process of being installed.

Martin and Jackie have developed a unique model in that The Exodus Project goes beyond dispensing services. They are keen to build up relationships with the whole family and not just the child that attends the mid- week clubs. In addition, once children have reached the age of fourteen, they are invited to help out with the younger groups as junior volunteers. Once they reach the age of eighteen, they become adult volunteers. This model provides a constant supply of help from individuals who have benefitted already from attending such groups.

The building is large and inviting. It is decorated with bold colours and has comfy seating. It is a real home from home; a haven for families who have been disadvantaged by the closure of the life force of its community.

Martin and Jackie have clear ideas about how they wish to develop the Exodus Project but the lottery funding which they benefitted from is no longer available. Sadly, they have had to close two of their clubs due to lack of funding. This decision wasn't taken lightly. They do have two charity shops which raises some money and they obtain some funding from outside organisations for the use of their facilities.

However, this is clearly not enough to keep their clubs, weekend activities   and building going to cater for the ever growing number of children who are benefitting from the work being undertaken here.   Neither does it allow for future development.

Exodus do have a Just Giving page which can be found here if you wish to help further their work https://www.justgiving.com/exodus

In addition, you can keep up with activities on their Facebook page here

https://www.facebook.com/search/top/?q=the%20exodus%20project%20barnsley&epa=SEARCH_BOX

Recommended small businesses

https://skinkiss.org.uk/

https://favouritekafei.co.uk/?fbclid=IwAR1pW2OJNWCtFdIpgU7WWp9JQiQDxbBxu4GfzBfr6648snFYFERRYvGW7Ss

Printed in Great Britain
by Amazon